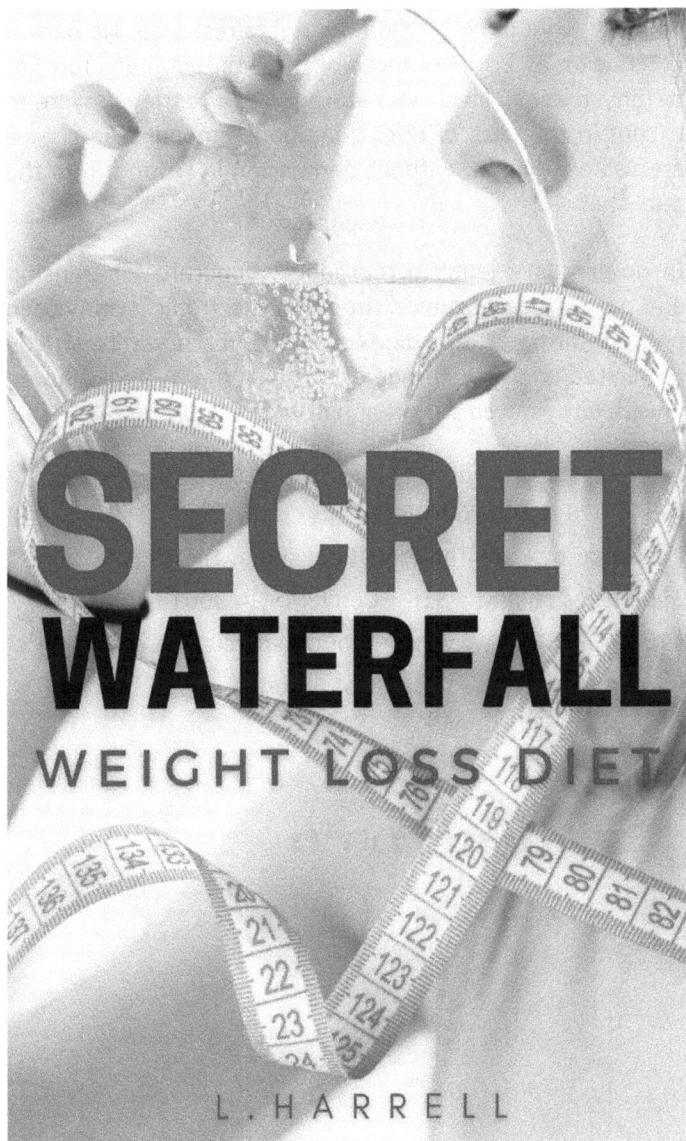

SECRET WATERFALL

WEIGHT LOSS DIET

L. HARRELL

Copyright © 2021 L. Harrell

ISBN: 978-1-953760-05-0

Published by Pure Thoughts Publishing, LLC

2055 Gees Mill Rd #316 | Conyers, GA 30013 USA

470-440-0875 | www.purethoughtspublishing.com

Printed in the United States of America

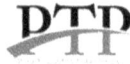

PTP

TABLE OF CONTENTS

INTRODUCTION

I'm writing this book because I struggle with my weight. I am currently 5'4 and 191 lbs. This is my experience from my personal point of view. My intentions are not to diagnose, treat you, nor am I an expert. Hopefully, this book will provide a glimmer of hope and help you to be encouraged along your weight loss journey. This is my honest testimony as to how I lost weight when all else had failed. I am a regular person just like you. I am a working single mother, a daughter, a sister, a best friend, a student of practical nursing, and a student of life. In this book, I will give you detailed information that you can use to lose those stubborn pounds that just will not budge once you have hit that plateau. I will tell you what to expect while water fasting. Your body will go through changes that you have never felt before. Your discipline will be put to the test in ways that you never thought it could be. Use water fasting as a way to jump-start your healthy new life. I personally never water fast for longs periods. My fasts are no more than 4 days, and I have still seen great results every time. What I have learned from doing this water fast several times, is the level of hunger that you will feel on day 1, will depend on how much food you eat the day before. For example, if you are like me, you will try and eat as much as you can the day before, knowing you will not have food for the next 4 days. This results in your body taking in a whole lot of calories. These calories are held in your body, which results in a fuller feeling on day 1, even though you haven't eaten anything. Also, I have learned to always reward myself before and after water fasting. It's necessary because that gratification is well deserved. Rewarding yourself also gives your body a break to get the nutrients that you will be depleted of. Taking a break also gives you time to reflect and plan your next fast. While reflecting on my reward days, I also think of ways to make the next fast better. While fasting, I'm usually full of energy and often I will feel the need to work out, but I do not. Rest is rest.

Another thing that you should think about is the fact that you will be hungry. You will lose the desire to socialize, especially when it involves food. You will see that eating is part of everything that we do. My family and friends did not see me the whole time. It's best that way so that I am not tempted by the smell of food. I did not want to hear any negative opinions or myths that would discourage me from completing the fast. You will see that the people that you love the most are the people who will try to change your mind or make you feel like you have an eating disorder.

Day 1

As soon as I woke up, I immediately drank one whole 16 oz bottle, which I keep on my nightstand just in case I'm not ready to get out of bed. That bottle of water helps to get the digestive system going. It also makes me feel full faster. I even do this when I'm not water fasting. After getting out of bed, I take a warm bath for relaxation. This also helps me to focus and get my mind prepared for the fact that I will not be eating for the rest of the day. You will see that a hot bath will become mandatory as your body loses its heat as each day goes by. I stopped at my local supermarket to shop for dinner for my son. Remember to feed your kids during this time. I usually still enjoy cooking dinner even though I cannot eat. My mouth started feeling extremely dry at about 10:30 am. I packed my Iron pill just in case I feel a little too weak. While at work, I catch myself yawning more than usual. I would still say that my energy level is normal. I keep looking at the clock to see how much time before

I go to lunch. I'm not concerned with eating, but more concerned with taking a nap. I went to lunch and sat in my car. I kept constantly fantasizing about crab legs with the special sauce from my favorite restaurant. I start watching my favorite show on my phone. This gives me something to focus on besides food. I tried to study for my nursing exam but I stopped because I could not focus. My job had the nerve to cater lunch, but I kindly declined. These are the things that will throw you off track. After I came back from lunch, I went to the restroom and looked at my tongue. It had the nastiest white film on it and my mouth tasted like death. My teeth are white.

- ➢ 6/9/2020 6:00 am Woke up at 7:30 am, Got to work

- ➢ 8:00 am Started feeling hungry 9:11 am, Dry mouth

- ➢ 9:37 am Yawning

- ➢ 10:30 am Food cravings,

- ➢ 11:30 am Lunch Break

- ➢ 12:30 pm Drank 3rd bottle of water

- ➢ 1:45 pm Felling a little tired

- ➢ 2:43 pm Yawning again

- ➢ 3:26 pm Bathroom break and feeling hungry 4:00 pm Feeling tired and hard to focus

- ➢ 5:30 am Not talking much and exhausted

- ➢ 7:30 pm Put water in the freezer and went to bed

- ➢ 12:30 am Woke up confused with horrible taste in my mouth

Day 2

It's day 2 and I woke up feeling surprisingly good. I drank my usual bottle of water. I am feeling optimistic about getting my day started and getting it over with. On day 2, I found myself thinking that I had made it one whole day without any food. This is a small milestone, but I am still proud of myself. If I quit now, I still accomplished something. I went to bed fairly early last night, which is unusual for me. I noticed that my body pretty much forced me to rest. I fell asleep slow and steady, but not exhausted. I slept well. The first few hours of work went smoothly. At about 10:00 am, I felt myself frowning uncontrollably. I'm not mad, but I cannot smile. I felt like I was rocking the resting bitch face. After lunch, I started getting sleepy and could not stop yawning, despite going to bed early. At the end of the workday, I felt sleepy, but still, alert. My eyes are straining and I could barely focus, but I'm still alert at the same time. I know it sounds confusing, but you are not yourself while water fasting. I went to bed at 9:30 pm. I could not sleep. I tossed and turned for hours. It's like I had reserved my energy. We use a lot of energy to digest food. Because I had no food to digest, my energy levels were unusually high, when I should have been preparing for bed. I woke up with night chills. My hands and feet were often cold. I had to sleep with a space heater pointed directly at me. I slept in thermal pajamas and 2 blankets. Yes, I was bone-chilling cold.

Day 3

Day 3 was interesting but yet productive. This is the day that I have heard most people say that the hunger pains go away. I noticed when I woke up on day 3, I did not feel hungry. I still had my usual bottle of water, but I did not feel the need to drink the whole bottle. I eventually drank it all, out of fear of being dehydrated. I had mucus in my throat on day 3 as well, which I kept spitting out the remainder of the day. Even though I woke up about 3 times at night, and did not sleep well, I was still full of energy with a positive outlook on life. My body felt lighter, which made me want to weigh myself. I didn't give in to the urge. I did my research about weighing in too often while trying to lose weight. We often make this mistake. You shouldn't weigh yourself every day, because our weight fluctuates from day-to-day. Everybody knows by now about the whole idea of a few pounds lost can be nothing more than water weight. I waited until the morning of the 5th day to weigh myself. I do not like false numbers. I remember one day I lost a pound after a hot bath. On this day, during my lunch break, I drank less water. I had normal energy. This day was a lot different from the previous days, where I wanted to take a nap. My hunger was not as bad as day 2, but I was still a little hungry off and on. At about 2:00 pm, my hands and arms started to get extremely cold. I had to grab a jacket to remain comfortable. My mouth was not as dry today. My eyes are extremely weak. My work computer screen was starting to become distorted where I could barely make out the words. By 3:15 pm, I became extremely sleepy and started dozing off. By 5:30, I got off of work. I raced to get in my car and prepare for the 45-minute dry home. I had to listen to satellite radio to keep myself awake during this slow boring moment. By 9:30 pm, I was in the bed, staring at the ceiling and anticipating my last day of water fasting. I couldn't help but think of how I felt, and if this was something that I could continue doing for the rest of my life. I slowly started to dismiss the bizarre rumors I had heard about water fasting. I went to bed on day 3 at 9:30 pm. My stomach was growling so bad that I could not stand it. I had to get up and walk around for a few minutes. I still could not get comfortable for the hunger pains. I woke up about 2 more times in the middle of the night.

- ➢ 5:30 am Woke up

- ➢ 7:30 am I have to work, energy level is alert, drank a bottle of water.

- ➢ 10:00 am My energy level is normal. I had 1 more bottle of water.

- ➢ 11:00 Lunch break. Normal energy. More energy than yesterday and had less water. 11:30 am came back from lunch and drank 1 more bottle of water.

- ➢ Noon arms and hands are cold

- ➢ 2:18 pm eyes are very weak. Ready to take a nap.

- ➢ 3:15 pm Mucus is in my throat.

Day 4

Day 4 is the best day of them all of course it's the last day of the fast and you're anticipating on eating your favorite foods. You're probably wondering why I chose to do a 4-day fast on the 4th day of water fasting your body goes into ketosis. This is when your body starts to burn fat the first three days your body fuels itself with carbohydrates I personally don't prefer to do more than 4 days based on my personal experience if you prefer to do so then that's great after 4 days I experienced dizziness fatigue anxiety muscle weakness and just an overall feeling of uneasiness doing during my fast I like to feel energized or at least level so that I can at least have enough energy to work out if I decide to do so after the fourth day I was too weak to work out.

➤ 5:50 am woke up

➤ 7:30 am got to work. My energy was low. I did not sleep well. Brushed my teeth and noticed a lot of mucus in my throat

➤ 8:41 am I am really hungry. Drank one bottle of water. I think today will be the hardest. it's early and I'm really hungry. I'm usually not this hungry until the end of the day or right before bed.

➤ I'm catching myself daydreaming

➤ 11:00 am lunchtime. I drank one bottle of water at 11:52 am energy is normal

➤ 1:17 pm yawning. My eyes are tired

➤ 3:00 pm tired of drinking water. My mouth tastes nasty 5:24 off work. Can't wait to get home

In this chapter I will discuss different pointers that helped me along the way of my fast. Let's be honest we all need that little push over the hump. Nobody's perfect and you will fall off from time to time. You may even break the fast and have to start all over again, but as long as you start over again then you're okay.

Pointer #1:

ind a social media support group. These groups are filled with people with the same goals as you and me. I connected with some individuals on these forums and you become each other's support system. You can bounce ideas off of each other or you can ask questions, chat, and share your experiences with each other as well. It's nothing like having a friend to talk to that's just a click away. It almost makes fasting more realistic when you see real people doing it too. This is one of the things that helped me on my recent fast. These support groups were not available when I first started fasting, so I definitely can appreciate them in modern times.

Pointer # 2

Find a hobby. Fasting can be very boring at times, so I suggest that you find something to keep your focus. Remember you will have a tremendous amount of extra time. You would not believe how much time we spend eating food. I found myself very bored, so I took the extra time that I had and helped my son with his homework. I also took walks in the park and j spent a lot of time reflecting on my life. I took this time to think about the goals that I would like to accomplish in life and what I would do once I completed the fast. I thought about my eating habits and what I would do to make healthier choices for me and my family. I prayed a lot because I am a spiritual being. I also took two courses that I needed to get into a nursing program. During this time that kept my focus where it needed to be.

Pointer #3

Preserve your energy. While fasting I also noticed that it took a tremendous amount of energy to do the simplest tasks. I often became winded while attempting to do normal everyday things. Things such as driving home from work seemed extra-long, climbing the stairs may seem impossible, and standing up to take a shower. Without a question, I suggest taking it easy on the 4th day. I became very weak and my mind will often go into a euphoric state. Limit yourself to brisk walking and light activity. Taking it easy was a hard part for me because I am usually active. There were times when I wanted to hit the gym and work out but I could not.

Pointer #4

Think of different ways to drink water. Drinking room-temperature water will eventually become boring to your taste buds. I found different ways to enjoy my water so that I could trick my mind into thinking that I was actually drinking something different. But in reality, it was all still water. For instance, I would freeze my water and make ice cubes. Sometimes I would warm my water up and imagine myself drinking warm tea. I always put my water on my nightstand before going to bed, it helps when you don't have to get up extra early just to walk down to the kitchen and make a glass of water. It's much easier when your water is at arm's reach. Especially when you wake up in the middle of the night and you're thirsty.

Pointer #5

Be sure that you are drinking enough water. I know there are some people out there who just do not like the taste of water. Therefore, on this type of fast, I would suggest that you be mindful that you are indeed taking in enough water. Remember the average human being can survive without food but we cannot survive without water. I tried to drink at least one whole gallon of water a day during my fast. Drinking more than a gallon of water a day caused my bladder to become weak, so proceed with caution. I try not to drink water after 9 p.m. to avoid interruptions in my sleep pattern.

Pointer #6

Don't tell people. I didn't tell people that I was water fasting, it just worked better for me if people did not give me their opinions about me only drinking water. I have done this fast several times and I have noticed that when you tell people that you are water fasting, they become concerned because of their own ignorance. They will think that you are starving yourself. People may also force you to eat. They will think that you are being extreme as if you are breaking the law or committing one of the forbidden Ten Commandments. I suggest you keep this a secret until you are finished.

Pointer#7

Do not weigh yourself throughout the water fast it will discourage you and make you want to quit. Remember, weighing yourself too early can give you false numbers. Water weight can be very misleading. I suggest you weigh yourself after day four when your body has begun to go through ketosis. That's when your body is using your fat for fuel. If you weigh yourself after ketosis the numbers on the scale are more likely to be true. I don't like to weigh myself often. I usually will weigh myself maybe once every two or three weeks, whether I'm water fasting or not. I just don't like to get false numbers. You don't want to get discouraged if the scale does not match the hard work that you have been putting in. I would not weigh myself until the morning of the end of the fast. During the four-day water fast, you would weigh in on the morning of the fifth day, do not eat before weigh-in. Try not to try to have a bowel movement if you can. Take a warm bath and get completely naked before weighing in. For some reason, I lost a pound after a warm bath.

Pointer #8

Don't sweat the small stuff. During water fasting, your mind must be clear of all stress. I know it's hard not to think of the everyday hustle and bustle that most of us have to go through to make a living, but I would suggest that you keep your stress level to a minimum. I've accomplished some of my longest water fast successfully when I was at my most peaceful moments in life. I know that there are always going to be stumbling blocks in the way that we just cannot avoid but try to keep your mental state clear of negativity. Some people like myself are just nervous by nature so I have to work hard to keep my peace. Sometimes this may be avoiding people that may bring extra stress into your life. Unfortunately, some of these people may be our family and our closest friends. It's okay to be away from these people for four days while you're trying to work on yourself. I'm sure they will understand.

About Author

L. Harrell studied to be a chiropractor at Life University because she was interested in a holistic approach to healing the body. She later served in the military where she learned how to use her mind over matter by adopting the core values necessary to survive as a soldier. During this time is when she started to experiment and learned that the human body can survive for long periods without food. After years of trial and error and being overweight, she has created a hassle-free method that will cost you nothing and keep you losing body fat. She resides in the Atlanta Metro area where she continues to practice her secret method.

You DON'T have to exercise or stress over calorie counting to LOSE WEIGHT!

Change your life today! Why wait until the new year to commit to a resolution? Treat your body to the waterfall weight loss method. Get a Head-start so you could be that much ahead of everyone else.

www.ingramcontent.com/pod-product-compliance
Lightning Source LLC
Chambersburg PA
CBHW070746280326
41934CB00011B/2815